Natural Antibiotics And Antivirals For Beginners

An Easy Guide To Herbal Medicine And Natural Healing

I0429957

Disclaimer

This book is intended to be a general guide, to raise awareness, and to help people make informed decisions in the context of their own personal circumstance. As everybody's circumstances are different, so are the remedies you should seek. While many of the recommendations in this book can be applied by almost anybody regardless of their conditions they are not intended to and should not be relied upon to replace personal medical advice.

The author accepts no responsibility for any loss or injury, be it personal or financial, as a result for the use or misuse of the information in this book. If you have any doubts or concerns after reading this book, please speak to a doctor or other qualified person before taking any actions.

From The Author

Thank you for taking the time to read this book. As an author, I understand the importance of creating books which my readers will find both enjoyable and informative. If you have the time and feel generous, please don't hesitate to leave an honest review of this book.........Dr Brad Turner.

TABLE OF CONTENTS

Introduction

The aim of this book is to give relevant, accurate and seriously researched information about the benefits of the medical herbs, specifically about the antibacterial and antiviral herbs.

In this book, we explain what you need to do to prepare and use the herbs to cure infectious diseases; we are going to take you to the times when our ancestors prepared their medicines using the herbs that were handy at nature, becoming experts in the way they must be prepared to give the best results.

In this world, where each day the prices of the antibacterial and antivirals go up because the pharmaceutical industry is colluded in a monopoly so they can charge for their products all they want; in this accelerated world of technology, of virtual relations, where is very easy to travel; in this world where the majority of the population is concentrated in the big cities, where nature has been invaded, destroyed or altered-- nature is every day farther away from our daily living.

We eat thousands of chemical products, such as colorants and preservatives, in our meals, and our medications have become completely synthetic; medicines have many secondary effects and contraindications. However, a lot of them are based on the herbology of our forefathers, the problem is that it is a synthetic herbology, with chemical substances added to preserve them and c.b.p excipient to compact them in a pill or capsule.

Those herbs that our ancestors used could be the solution to our infectious diseases where traditional medicine works with synthetic drugs, or sometimes, it does not work at all. We have developed many bacterial resistances-- here is where the mystic and magic herbology of our ancestors will help us.

We invite you to delve into the pages of this book, where the wonderful world of herbology that maintained the health of our antecessors will help you to acquire the knowledge of the antibiotic and antiviral herbs that have been recovered from the past, and that for the word has come to us to be rescued.

Actually, these herbs have been completely researched to prove their efficacy and to know the contraindications, so much that pharmaceutical laboratories are using them to produce their synthetic medicines.

Following very simple steps, you will be able to prepare them exactly as needed to give their maximum force and to help you cure the infectious diseases with natural products.

Let us introduce you to the fascinating world of the antimicrobial and antiviral herbs.

Chapter 1

Antibiotic And Antiviral Herb Overview

Many herbs have medicinal or tonic value, and many times are mixed into meals to prevent or treat common diseases. Traditional therapies typically use herbs as medicines and many pharmaceuticals are derived from herbs and other plants. Herbs have provided a blueprint for most modern drugs.

And the nature has not changed. Humans evolved in a plant environment and were shaped and conditioned by it, and humans survived in part thanks to what plants gave them, especially when they were ill, and humans acquired the knowledge of the natural pharmacy. All the plants held a key for some ailment, either in its natural state, mixed with others, or after distillation.

Ancient and traditional stories about the medical effects of herbs are glutted with magic and superstition-- and that is why herbal lore got a bad name in the sixteenth century.

But these days, all plants have been proven at the laboratories, and substances like salicylic acid are more effective than the salicylic acid derived from the willow, the predecessor of aspirin, but science has sunk the findings of the past, tested through thousands of years of use with such care that no laboratory program can afford.

All those centuries of testing in people now are replaced by three or four months of testing in laboratory rats or guinea pigs. Long term effects cannot be known; meanwhile, wild flowers bloom and die naturally, their offers refused and their powers to heal ignored.

Lately, herbs have regained popularity and are being used again; people are using herbs again to keep their health and to cure diseases, and antibiotic and antiviral herbs are some of the most used because of their good results.

Herbal medicine uses parts of plants or their essential oils; they can be used as an infusion, in the form of tea, as a cataplasm, creams, tinctures, decoctions and hydrodistillation.

Before using plant based remedies, it's important that you know exactly how to prepare them and which contraindications or secondary effects they have, to be sure you won't have any negative side effects.

Chapter 2

Antibacterial Herbs And How To Use Them

Basil

(Ocimum basilicum L.)

The volatile oils of basil limonene have shown the potential to protect against bacterial growth, like strains of some gram positive bacteria, but most of these bacteria are gram-negative bacteria that infect the 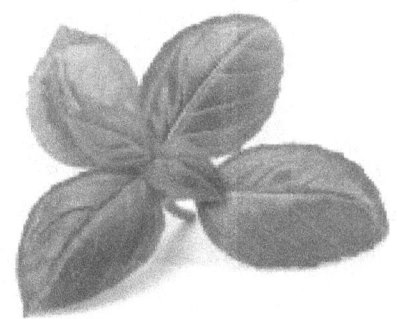 digestive system, producing among others diarrhea. These bacteria have shown antibiotic resistance, but they are controlled by the essential oil that is obtained from the basil leaves, where all the antioxidants and essential volatile oils are stored.

The way to obtain basil protection benefits against bacteria is by eating it in meals; to receive the cure benefits you need to hydrodistillation, which is the official standard method for extracting essential oils for quality control. At home it is made by just boiling the leaves in hot water and then passing them in a strainer to collect the water with all the essential oils. Drink this infusion every 8 hours until diarrhea disappears.

Basil does not have any known secondary effects or contraindications.

Cayenne Pepper

(Capsicum annum, Capsicum minimum or Capsicum frutescents)

Its antibacterial activity is due to the increased immunity that it provides, because it has high levels of vitamins, like vitamin A, which has a very powerful anti-bacterial effect.

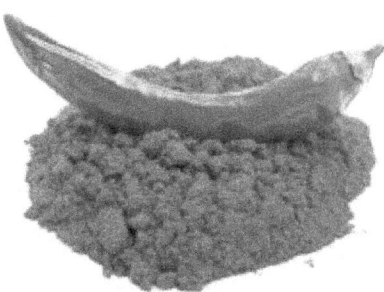

Also, it works to clear lung and respiratory tract congestion, and by doing this, it prevents bacterial infections.

To obtain these benefits, one must take 30 to 120 mg of cayenne pepper one to three times a day. Boil some water and add a half teaspoon of cayenne pepper; drink it 3 times a day.

Important- People with digestive disease must avoid taking cayenne pepper because it produces a higher quantity of acid and may cause abdominal pain, bleeding, and anemia.

Eyes and skin contact should be avoided because it is very irritating for them.

Cayenne pepper may cause allergic reactions that go from mild ones to anaphylactic shock; people that have allergies to latex, chestnuts, banana, kiwi, or avocado are more prone to be allergic to cayenne pepper

Cinnamon

(Cinnamomum verum)

It owes its antibacterial properties to essential oils; it has been proven to have antibacterial activity against gram negative bacteria and antifungal activity against candida albicans and other fungi.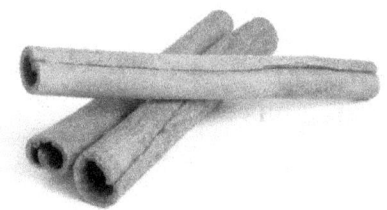

If you inhale the essential oil of cinnamon, you will clean your respiratory system and will be able to stay free of irritation and cough caused by respiratory bacteria.

Prepare it by adding 5 drops of the cinnamon oil into a bowl of boiling water, and just breathe over it. Be careful not to get too close and burn your face with the steam.

Cinnamon can be taken as a tea, three cups a day to treat cold symptoms.

Important- Do not use during pregnancy, especially in the last months, because it is a uterine stimulant.

If you take blood thinning medication, avoid cinnamon, because it thins the blood too.

Comfrey roots

(Symphytum officinale)

The antibacterial properties of the Comfrey come from its antioxidants and its acids that have been widely used for bacterial diseases of the upper respiratory tract.

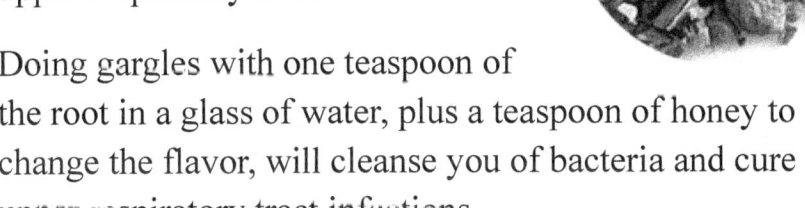

Doing gargles with one teaspoon of the root in a glass of water, plus a teaspoon of honey to change the flavor, will cleanse you of bacteria and cure upper respiratory tract infections.

It is used to treat bronchitis and is an expectorant.

Also, it can be used for uterine infections or inflammation of the uterine walls; it must be used as irrigations do with the hydrodistillation product of the root.

It has mucilage, and it helps to shoot mucous ulcers at the stomach and gut. It has an astringent property that reduces bleeding

For internal use, do decoctions. These are made by taking 1 to 3 teaspoons of dried extract and boiling it in 30 ounces of water for 20 minutes. After that, pass it through a strainer and take one cup three times a day.

Important- The plant is used in this way, but it has toxic compounds, so even though it sometimes is used for internal derangements, we recommend using it only for gargles or uterine irrigations.

Mallows

(Althaea officinalis)

As an antibacterial, it is widely used to treat bronchitis, but it is also used as an expectorant. In 30 ounces of water, put 100grms of the dry roots, wait until it boils, and then pass it through a strainer and add 3 pounds of sugar. Take half of a little glass of this syrup at night time before going to bed.

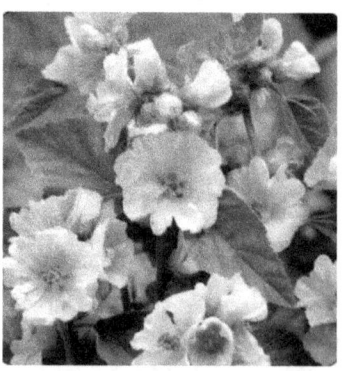

Chronic bladder infections respond particularly well to mallow preparations, and it helps to avoid repeated antibiotic

therapy. Make a hydrodistillation with the dry roots of the plant and drink 3 to 5 cups of tea each day until your symptoms lower, then you can use only one cup a day.

There have not been adverse effects reported of marshmallow herb.

Myrrh

(Commiphora myrrha)

This stimulates the circulation of mucosal tissue. It has antibacterial, anti-inflammatory and antioxidant properties that make it the ideal herb to treat mouth and throat infections, plus bronchitis.

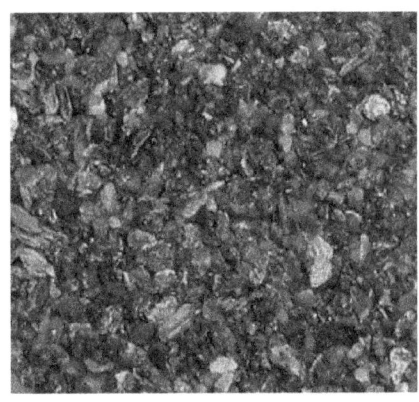

Myrrh is not well diluted in water, so it is used as a tincture; it is typically made with 1 part of myrrh for 5 parts of 90-% ethanol and 10-% water. Use 5 to 10 drops of this tincture and add 8 ounces of water to it; now it is ready to be used for a mouthwash or gargle. The tincture can be applied directly to sore gums.

The diluted tincture can be used over skin infections or irrigated for vaginal infections.

You can find myrrh capsules in the herbal stores. One capsule of 200 mg 5 times a day substitutes the infusion for internal usage to treat bronchitis.

Important- Myrrh is contraindicated in pregnant women because it has tightening effects on the uterus muscles.

If you have any heart condition or diabetes, you should consult a physician first.

A safe dose of myrrh is less than 2,000mgs a day, do not overdose.

Chapter 3

Antiviral Herbs And How To Use Them

Calendula

(Calendula officinalis)

Known as garden marigold, marigold, or gold bloom.

It has been used since the 12th century and is produced in tinctures,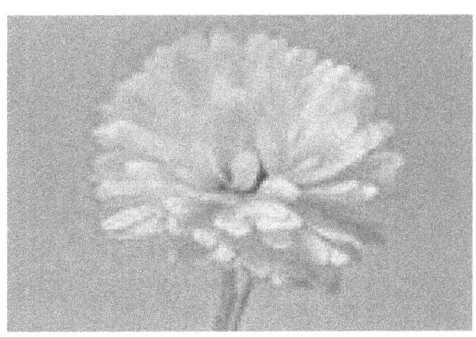
infusions, lotions, ointments and extracts.

It is used to promote wound healing, reduce inflammation, and to prevent soft tissue infection.

To prepare the infusion, you need two teaspoons of dried flowers and two cups of hot water. Let it simmer for 10 minutes and pass it through a strainer. Drink it 3 times a day.

There are not side effects or contraindications known.

Cranberry

(Vaccinium oxycoccos)

This is an excellent herb in preventing urinary infections; it changes the bladder lining so microorganisms can stick to it. Cranberry has antiviral properties and also oxidant properties.

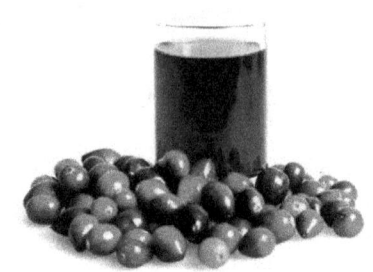

Use it as unsweetened juice or in tablets, 2 tablets 3 times a day. Or 3 glasses of juice per day.

Important- Don't use in predisposition to kidney disease or pregnancy or lactation. More than 3 to 4 L a day may produce gastrointestinal symptoms such as diarrhea. Concentrated tablets may predispose to kidney stone formation.

Echinacea

(Echinacea angustifolium)

It was used to prevent infection in venomous bites (mosquito, snake, scorpion, wasp, others).

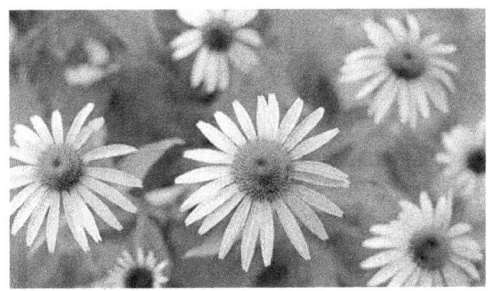

It was used to reduce pain and infection in any kind of wound.

It was used as a pain killer and healer for burns.

Today is used to treat cold and influenza symptoms. It has been rediscovered and is used to treat fungal and viral infections; it has been used in AIDS treatments.

It works to boost the immune system and its response to viral infections is helpful.

That is why you may take an Echinacea tincture to prevent or treat a cold and your immune system will do the rest.

You can buy tincture or capsules at the herbal store; the tea has a very bad taste.

For acute infections it is recommended you take one teaspoon of tincture every 3 hours. You may also take 6 capsules a day divided into 3 doses, one each 8 hours.

If you have a chronic infection then you must prolong the treatment, same as your physician would do if you were taking pharmaceutical medicine; so take half teaspoon of tincture or 2 capsules 4 times a day for 3 weeks, then rest for about 6 weeks and take it all over again.

<u>Important</u>- Some people may be allergic to the herb, especially those that are allergic to ragweed.

Elderberry

(Sambucus nigra)

The flowers and the berries have anti-inflammatory properties and are used to calm a sore throat, cough, bronchial infection, and sinus 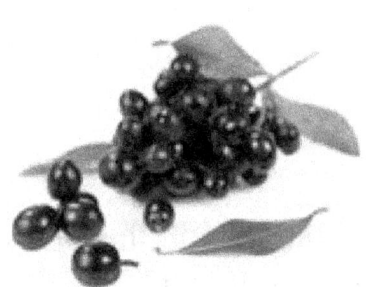 congestion. It is a very effective antiviral herb used to treat colds, flu, and also help to prevent them. It also has antioxidant potential.

Usually, it is taken as elderberry syrup, the dose 15ml taken 4 times a day, every day until infection symptoms disappear.

There are not contraindications or side effects known.

Important- Consumption of uncooked berries may result in diarrhea and vomiting.

Eucalyptus

(Eucalyptus Globus)

The leaves of the tree are the ones that are used to do its primary function: move mucous secretions. That is what gives eucalyptus is power over viral diseases of the respiratory tract, cough, asthma, bronchitis, pneumonia, and tuberculosis.

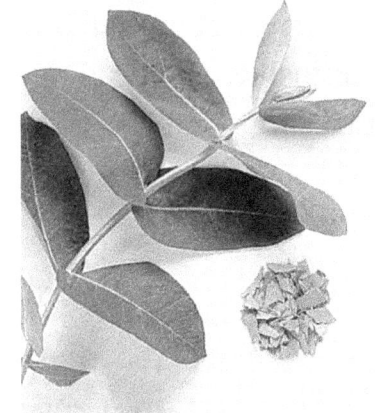

In a steamer, you put 30 ounces of water plus 5 drops of the essential eucalyptus oil and inhale, which will move all the obstructions out of the system, relieving the cold and flu symptoms.

The fresh leaves can be used to make a tea or gargles for bronchitis, sinusitis, and a sore throat.

For external use it has to be mixed, 10 to 20 drops into half a cup of almond oil, and then you can use it on your skin.

Important- Eucalyptus essential oil is very strong and should not be used without dilution.

It may burn your skin if used undiluted.

You should never eat or drink it without dilution; it can burn your insides and result in death. Always follow dilution instructions and don't leave it within reach of children.

Lemon Balm

(Mellissa officinalis)

It has calming properties and it is used to treat stress and anxiety.

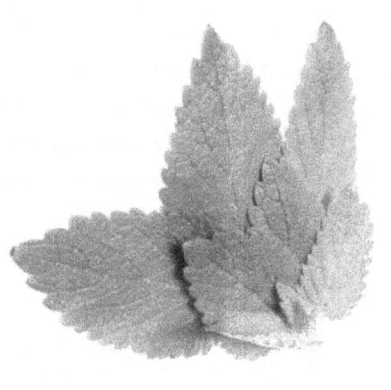

It is a member of the mint family and is delightful; the leaves contain an essential oil which gives the herb its antiviral properties.

It can be used to treat colds and cold sores.

It is used to treat herpes simplex virus, especially the one that appears between the skin and the mouth vermillion; it is particularly useful to smooth the lips.

You can find the essential oil at the herbalist stores and you can make the tea.

Use a quarter of a cup of fresh lemon balm leaves and a cup of water, boil it for a minute, and then leave it covered for 5 minutes. The tea will be ready with a delicious aroma; take 3 cups a day until herpes disappears.

There are no reports of secondary effects or contraindications.

Licorice

(Glycyrrhiza glabra)

It works very wellfor healing coughs, inflammation, stomach ulcers, canker sores, and cold sores produced by herpes simplex virus. It is used to treat flu, herpes, and 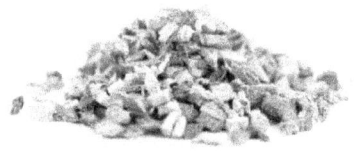 hepatitis virus. It is said that it may suppress HIV activity and can be helpful for AIDS patients. Licorice enhances mucosal protection and is better than any antacid.

Licorice is used to treat inflammation of the lungs, bowels, and skin. It mimics the activity of cortisol, a natural hormone of our body, and that is why it has such an anti-inflammatory action.

Licorice is also antioxidant, antispasmodic, and expectorant.

Licorice may be purchased dried, as tinctures and capsules, also as elixir and syrups.

To treat stomach ulcers or irritable bowel episodes, the dose is 3 to 4 cups a day, prepared as a tea.

Pour boiling water over the licorice root; keep it boiling for 10 minutes to obtain all the root components, pass it through a strainer, and drink it as a tea.

Important- May cause weight gain, fluid retentions, and hypertension. Do not use in pregnant women.

Tea Tree Oil

(Melaleuca alternifolia)

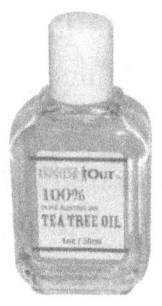

This is a good antiviral at nose level and as a nasal cream in a concentration of 4% applied each 8 hours for 5 days; as an antifungal and antibacterial agent, it works very hard to treat bacteria. It is used to treat fungi on the nails by applying tea tree oil at 100% for 6 months, and is used for athlete's foot with the tea tree oil at 50% for 6 months.

Important- Never use for oral ingestion. Do not use in pregnant women. It can produce dermal irritation in sensitive people.

Chapter 4

Herbs With Antibacterial And Antiviral Properties And How To Use Them

Cat's Claw

(Uncaria Tomentosa)

It has been used in Peruvian medicine to treat digestive complaints, arthritis, and to treat wounds, but most recently it is used to stimulate the immune system because of a compound it has that acts as an antioxidant and cleans the body of free radicals.

Some compounds found in Cat's claw are responsible for its effect to kill viruses and bacteria and helping healthy cells to avoid transforming into malignant ones.

It is used for herpes zoster virus, for cold sores caused by herpes simplex, and for AIDS caused by immunodeficiency virus.

Cat's Claw is taken as a tea, tincture, or capsule.

To make a tea if you use it ground, use 1 to 2 teaspoons in a tea strainer and then into a cup of boiling water. If you use bark, add one average piece to the boiling water.

If you add some lemon drops, it help to release the tannins of the tea. Let it sit for 10 minutes and remove the tea strainer. Add some spices or honey to make it more palatable.

Important- side effects could be dizziness, headache, and nausea.

Contraindicated in people with organ transplants

Contraindicated within two weeks before or after any type of surgery or for people with bleeding disorders.

Do not use in pregnant women or in children.

Garlic

(Allium sativum)

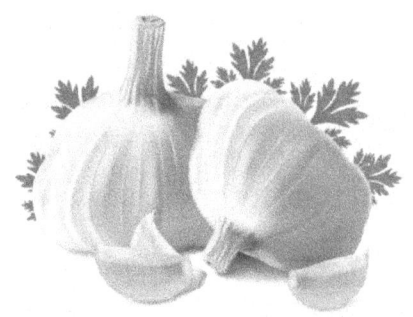

Bulb contains antibiotic substances; it is an immune system stimulant, due to its compounds. It has many properties, but as an antibacterial it is useful in diarrhea and other stomach troubles, is very good against worms, and kills bacteria in the digestive system, without harming the normal microbiota of the bowel. It is also very good for relieving viral infections of the respiratory tract and in preventing the flu, sinus disease, and bronchial congestion.

It can be taken raw, labored, as essential oil, tablets and capsules, inhaled, or applied directly to the affected parts. Most people don't want to smell like garlic, so it's easier to take it as tablets or capsules that you can buy at the drugstore or herbal store, but this is more expensive than the fresh bulb of garlic. You can always chew some fresh parsley after the garlic and it will take the odor away.

Start with a small amount of raw garlic because it can upset the stomach; 1/4 teaspoon 3 times a day, or if you choose to take capsules take one each 8 hours.

To prevent digestive system infections, cook your foods with garlic.

Important- if you are taking blood thinning medications, consult your medical doctor before using garlic.

Ginger

(Zingiber officinale)

Ginger has been used to treat digestive affections, stimulate the pancreas, and the enzyme production helps digestion, plus its antibacterial power is very useful in treating a wide range of intestinal diseases 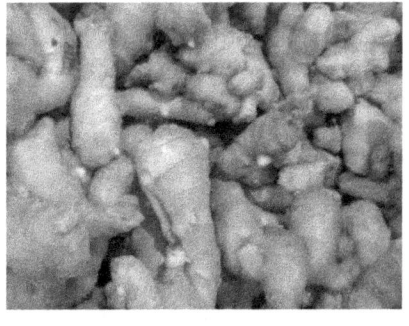 that produce alterations of the normal flora.

To treat ulcers at the digestive system that come for the presence of bacteria responsible for the ulcers, you can take it as an infusion; make a decoction with one spoon of ginger and let it stay for 2 hours, then pass it through a strainer and drink it as a tea each 8 hours until symptoms are gone.

It is very useful for treating diarrhea. It kills bacteria and parasites, helping the movement and restoring the health of the digestive system.

When using to treat cold symptoms, helping to expectorate, to relieve sinusitis congestion because of its action against viruses, or lowering fever and nasal congestion, take as an infusion with one spoon of dried root in a glass of water and when it is done add some lime juice to potentiate the effect with the C vitamin of the lime. Take it three times a day.

If using essential oil instead of decoction, use 9 drops divided into 3 doses of 3 drops every 8 hours, per day. Put the drops in a glass of water and drinks it. If using dry, extract 400mg split in 3 doses, one each 8 hours, per day, make an infusion with the extract and use it as a tea.

Important- if you take more than these doses, it can be toxic.

The maximum amount of fresh ginger you should take is 2gr. a day.

Goldenseal

(Hydrastis Canadensis)

This is a potent antibacterial and mild anti-inflammatory herb. It has astringent properties that make it useful for a swollen or infected throat, stomach, or vagina because it acts over the mucous membrane surface.

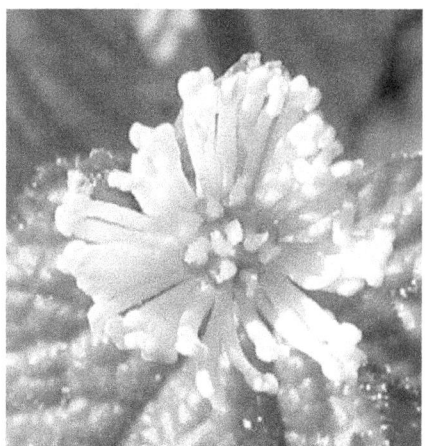

It is a miracle herb; for centuries it has been used for almost everything.

As an antibacterial herb, it is used to treat different diseases caused by bacteria; you can use the goldenseal in capsules that are sold at pharmacies.

To use it for external infections, do a decoction of the herb that you can buy at the pharmacy and follow their doses.

It is effective against skin infections, so it is used as a poultice over wounds of the skin.

For infected throat or oral sores, do gargles with the decoction 3 times a day.

For vaginal infections, do infusions of the decoction three times a day.

Effective for eye infections; use the same decoction only you need to wait until the decoction is cold.

Useful for urinary infections, too; take a cup of decoction 3 times a day.

Important- Should be avoided in pregnant women and during lactation.

Don't use it in kids under 15 years old because of its toxic contents.

Do not use it if you have hypertension, any heart condition, glaucoma, diabetes, or any immune disease.

If you are taking any pharmaceutical medication, consult your physician before taking goldenseal; it is contraindicated if you are taking any pharmaceutical drug.

Oregano

(Origanum vulgare)

It has antiviral effects against the cold and the flu, treats bacterial or viral pneumonia and bronchitis, boosts the immune system, and has decongestant activity; the oregano

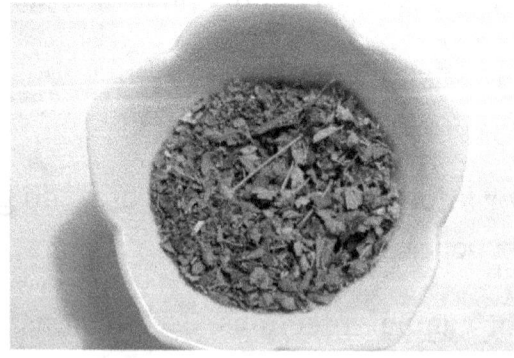

essential oils are high in antioxidants, and that gives the plant its antimicrobial activity. There are reports saying it kills almost all the gram negative bacteria, and also parasites like Giardia and athlete's foot

It has multiple actions is anti-inflammatory, antibacterial, antiseptic, antiviral, and antifungal, so some people refer to it as the strongest antimicrobial herb.

To use it for a throat sore, use one drop of essential oregano oil in a glass of water and do gargles. For coughing, put one drop into a small glass of water and drink it.

For athlete's foot, put your feet in a basin with water and two teaspoons of oregano essential oil or rub the oil through your feet.

Put some drops of oregano in a bowl and put it to boil; do inhalations for sinus or cold infections.

Put a drop of oregano oil in two spoons of water, put it in your mouth, and keep it there for a minute, then just swallow it. Do this four times a day to treat parasites.

Important- Oregano, as any other substance, may cause allergies. There have been some reports about oregano allergies, so if you are allergic to oregano or any plant of the same family: sage, basil, marjoram, lavender, or hyssop, don't use oregano at all.

Oregon grape

(Mahonia aquifolium)

Its preparations are used for infections and to improve liver function and digestion.

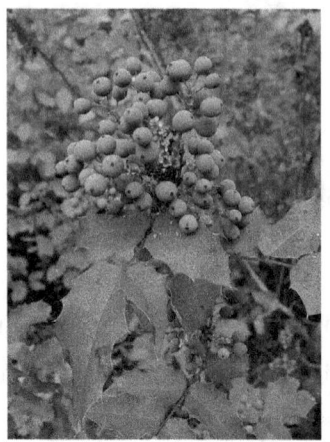

It is used to treat the cold, flu, and infections caused by bacteria and viruses.

There are many gram negative bacteria and parasites that are sensitive to the herb.

It is recommended for a vaginal douche, topically over the skin, as a tincture for different diseases of the skin.

Oregon grape is bitter so prepare the tea infusion by adding some orange peel or licorice into it. Drink 3 to 6 cups a day on the onset of infection and then reduce it until you are symptom free.

You may use capsules; take 2 capsules 3 to 4 times a day.

You could use the tincture, half a teaspoon every four hours for acute infection, and decreasing use with the decrease of symptoms.

Important- It has compounds that can be toxic, so restrict its use to 6 weeks; stop several weeks and then you can use it again if necessary. Do not use in pregnant women.

Peppermint

(Mentha piperita)

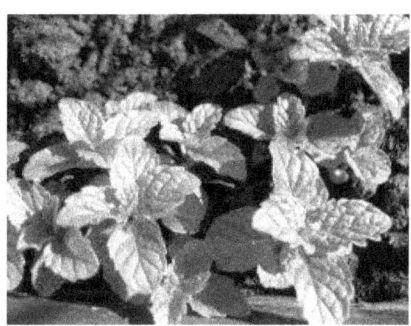

It has a lot of properties, between them being antibacterial and antiviral properties. It is used to treat tuberculosis; it regresses tuberculosis inflammation and prevents recurrence.

It helps to inhibit herpes virus simplex. It has an acid which helps to reduce inflammation in asthma patients.

It acts as an expectorant and decongestant of the respiratory tract, and relieves cold symptoms.

It has been found that it is better than some oral mouthwashes in preventing the formation of dental plaque, which is full of bacteria.

It works to treat headaches, stress, and alleviates muscle pain.

You can buy the essential oil, which you can use in your food to flavor it; also, you can put 2 drops in water to make your own mouthwash. Use it for herpes simplex mouth infection.

You can make a tea with the green leaves, the upper ones in the plant, by using a handful of leaves in boiling water; let it simmer 10 minutes and strain it.

Drink it 3 or 4 times a day until cold symptoms disappear; use it as a tea to treat lip herpes simplex virus.

Important- It can worsen hiatal hernia and worsen gallstones. If taking it too concentrated, it can cause ulcers in the mouth, and as with any drug or food, allergic reactions can occur.

Red Clover

(Trifolium pretense)

The flowers are the ones that are used for medical purposes.

To make the tincture, you need 8 ounces of dry blossoms in one pint of alcohol 50%. Take 1 to 10 drops as a dose.

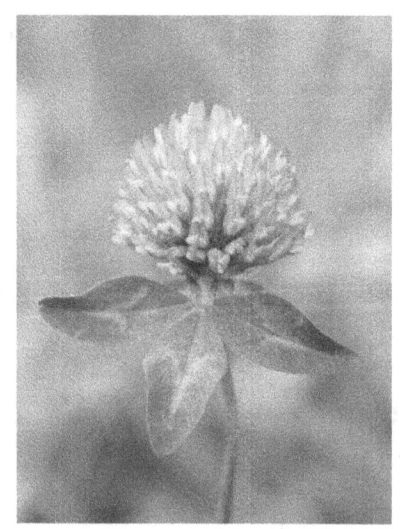

To make tea, use 480 grams in one ounce of fluid alcohol 30%. Use 10 drops to 1 gram in 4 ounces of water and take a teaspoon every 3 hours.

The herb is used to increase resistance to bacterial and viral infection, and it has proven to be effective against fungal infection, some parasites, and gram negative bacteria. This herb has amazing properties in addition to its viral and antibiotic properties.

Used as directed. It does not have side effects.

Sage

(Salvia officinalis)

A member of the mint family, it has strong antiseptic and antiviral properties and is an excellent decongestant for the respiratory diseases such as a cold, flu, and bronchitis. It is the principal remedy for threatening bacterial and viral infections and also has anti-inflammatory effects. It has been considered an herb to cure all.

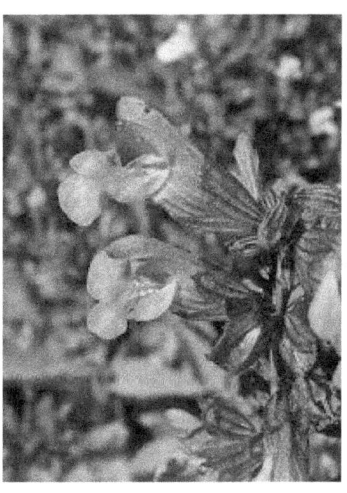

Is also can be used to treat mouth sores, canker sores, and a sore throat.

It can be used as a tea, prepared as syrup, or as an extract. It's bitter taste will go away with a little sugar or honey addition.

To make the tea, use a bunch of fresh sage leaves in 30 ounces of water, let it boil for 5 minutes, and pass through a strainer. Drink 3 to 4 times a day.

To make the syrup, use 1 cup of tea and 1 cup of sugar; let it boil until the sugar is integrated. You can also use fresh sage leaves and cover them with honey, let it simmer for an hour, and pass it through a strainer. Take 1 teaspoon as needed to treat a sore throat and mouth sores.

The extract can be made using the fresh leaves in decoction with half 15 ounces of water half a bunch of fresh leaves; leave them to boil until the water has reduce to almost half of the volume and pass it through a strainer-- that is the extract. Use 1 to 10 drops as a dose 3 times a day.

Important- Do not use if you are taking sedatives, due to the increased sedative effects. It may produce headaches, an upset stomach, restlessness, dizziness, and irritability.

Do not use in pregnant women or during lactation.

Yarrow

(Achillea millefolium)

It is used to treat infections and heal wounds; it acts as an immune stimulant. Another use is to reduce cold or flu symptoms.

To fight infection, it needs to be used 3 times a day until the infection is over.

To prevent infection, it should be used for one week.

To heal a wound, it must be packed into the wound 3 times a day.

Use one teaspoon of dried yarrow in one cup of boiling water.

Tincture in 1:5 dilution use 5ml= one teaspoon

Tincture diluted 1:1 use 20 drops

You may find it in capsules, essential oil, tincture, and dried at the herbal stores

It does not have known toxicity.

Important- Don't use in pregnant women.

Buying Or Growing Your Herbs

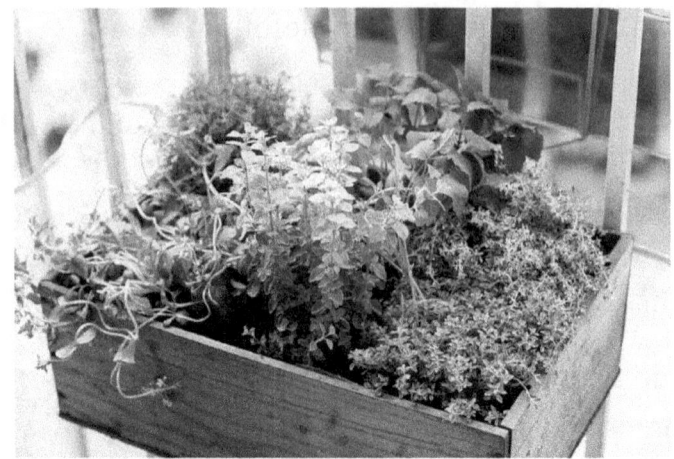

When it comes to starting to use herbs as medical remedies, you should ask yourself if you are going to use them once in a while or if you are going to use them routinely.

If you are looking to just use them once in a while, then it would be wiser to go to the herb store or a pharmacy when you need it, buy what you need, and when you are done with it, get rid of what is left, so you don't have old herbs in your house.

If you are going to integrate them into your way of life, then it would be a lot better to grow your own herbs. This way, you will always have handy whatever you need for you medical issues, but also, you will have a lot of fragrance and possibilities to add them to your foods in order to prevent diseases, even if you are absolutely healthy; some of them taste very good. And gardening, if you have the time, could be a great pastime.

There are 5 herbs that are easy to grow and can cover almost all of your needs. Of course, if you have a specific medical issue, you must add the specific herb to treat it, but to start a garden we recommend:

Peppermint is used especially as a digestive aid.

But it is known that its oil contains substances that inhibit the growth of bacteria and viruses; its primary compound is menthol and is also used for cramps, diarrhea, and nausea.

It's better to grow it in containers. It is very invasive; it needs moist, well-drained soil and full sun. You must harvest the leaves and dry them in a warm and dark place.

Make a delicious medical tea with 1 teaspoon of dry leaves and a cup of boiling water, let it sit 10 minutes, and strain it to your cup. Take 3 cups a day to help digestion.

Chamomile is good for easing digestion, relieving urinary colic, and other issues already discussed.

The flowers usually appear 6 weeks after planting them. It does well in sandy, well-drained ground, and it grows better in cool climates. It reproduces itself very easily so you can harvest the flowers and let them dry in a warm and dark place.

Now you are ready to make some tea. Just use a half teaspoon of dry flower and add boiling water, a cup, let it sit for 10 minutes, and strain into your cup. Take 4 cups a day if you have an upset stomach or one at nighttime as a relaxant for a good night's sleep.

Yarrow as seen previously, is excellent for stopping bleeding wounds and helps to heal them.

Plants are easily grown from seed or you can buy it already grown; it adapts well to every soil type. Plant in half shade and harvest the stalks when in full bloom; dry them in a warm, dark place by hanging them downwards.

If you cut yourself, just crush some leaves or flowers and apply them after washing the wound; bleeding will stop immediately.

You may also do a tea for stopping the cold and treat early fever; put 1 teaspoon of dry flowers or leaves into boiling water, wait 10 minutes for it to sit, and then strain into your cup. Drink it 3 times a day until symptoms disappear.

Echinacea In the previous chapter, you can read about its medicinal properties. Just remember, it's an excellent Immune-booster. You may have a little difficulty finding plants and seed of the E. angustifolia, which is the best kind for medical remedies. Look into seed houses and nurseries and you will find them. If you can't find them, you can try ordering them.

It grows well in any garden soil if it has a good drainage; it needs only half shade.

When it has flowers, you just need to put them under boiling water, and during the winter you may do a tincture. Chop the quantity of plant to use and mix it with proof grain alcohol, like half the bottle, and then a quarter of water. Cover it well and let it sit for 2 weeks. After this, you will have the tincture and you can use from 30 to 40 drops, 4 times a day, when you feel like you're catching a cold.

Lemon Balm works, as we said before, for a number of diseases and also to calm anxiety.

It grows easily from seeds during spring time, requires moist soil, and it grows better under shade; it needs to be pruned frequently, as it tends to invade.

It is better when used fresh because it retains its flavor this way. Make a tea with a handful of fresh leaves and boiling water. Drink it 3 times a day to treat any medical condition, or just to enjoy it.

With these advices, you are ready to start a pot garden, a garden in a patio, or even to have an herb garden itself, and you are ready to buy just what you need, when you need it. It all depends on your time and preferences.

Conclusion

With all the things that we know after reading this book, we are able to change the way we heal ourselves. We can stop taking pharmaceutical medications for a cold, or the flu, or even for a headache. In this way, our body will have less harmful chemicals inside and will be able to clean itself easier, leaving no residue of chemical drugs.

We are now capable of finding a great way to prevent diseases, that before were didn't know of, like if we take tea to prevent the flu at the first symptoms, instead of waiting to feel bad to go to the physician.

Now we have the possibility to grow an herbal garden that will fill the air with wonderful fragrances and that will be a great pastime.

And with the book, we have a very useful guide to use any time needed, using the different possibilities that this book has brought to us.

References

1.-Duman AD1, Telci I, Dayisoylu KS, Digrak M, Demirtas I, Alma MH. Antimicrobial action of essential oils: the effect of dimethylsulphoxide on the activity of cinnamon oilP. Hili2, C. S. Evans1 and R. G. Veness1Article first published online: 31 OCT 2003; DOI: 10.1046/j.1472-765X.1997.00073.x The Society for Applied Bacteriology 1997.

2. -"Forgotten" ingredients - Food Habits. (n.d.). Retrieved from http://foodhabits.eu/wp-content/results/Forgotten_ingredients_final.pdf (Consulted 26 July 2014.)

3. - HowStuffWorks "Oregon Grape: Herbal Remedies". (n.d.). Retrieved from http://health.howstuffworks.com/wellness/natural-medicine/herbal-remedies/oregon -grape-herbal-remedies.htm.

4.- J Agric Food Chem. 2003 May 21;51(11):3197-207.Antimicrobial properties of basil and its possible application in food packaging.Suppakul P1, Miltz J, Sonneveld K, Bigger SW. Glenn, Reschke. Learn About The Specific Health Benefits of Cayenne Pepper & How It Can Help You; 2007-2014 Copyright © www.CayennePepper.info.

5.- Salinas Sánchez David O., Arteaga Najera Gema L., León Rivera Ismael, Dorado Ramírez Oscar, Valladares Cisneros Ma. Guadalupe, Navarro García Víctor M... Antimicrobial activity of medicinal plants from the Huautla Sierra Biosphere Reserve in Morelos (Mexico). Polibotánica [revista en la Internet]. 2009 Sep [citado 2014 Jul 27]; (28): 213-225. Disponible en: http://www.scielo.org.mx/scielo.php?script=sci_arttext&pid=S1405-27682009000200010&lng=es.

Other Books By Dr Brad Turner

Headache Cures Made Easy

Headaches are extremely common, especially in today's society where everyone is stressed, exhausted and forever taking on too much work. However, the big problem arises when we stop viewing headaches as something serious. Whether large or small, headaches can often be a symptom of a more severe underlying problem and ignoring them is the worst thing we can do. Whether you regularly experience primary or secondary headaches, you can use this guide to learn about the causes of headaches, the symptoms that can 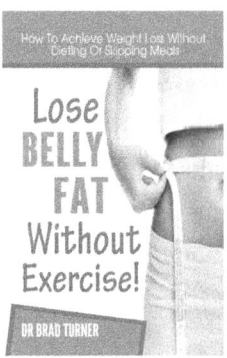 arise and how to tackle them if they are a common occurrence in your life. It also offers you details of natural cures, giving you useful tips and ideas to help stop that headache in its tracks, as well as information on how to prevent getting headaches and migraines in the future.

Lose Belly Fat Without Exercise

Dr Brad Turner's *Lose Belly Fat Without Exercise is* an easy to follow guide which gives you the important information you need to give you a jump start to a vibrant, radiant and sexy new you!

If you are tired of counting calories, fat grams and points and or have lost your motivation with crash course exercise programs and are tired of diets that just do not work, then this book is for you.

Aromatherapy The Beginner's Guide

Frankincense. Peppermint. Eucalyptus. Lemon-grass. Lavender. Who knew that these are five must-have essential oils? Dr. Brad Turner does—and we are blessed that he's chosen to share his knowledge and expertise in his latest book, ESSENTIAL OILS. So much has been written about using oils: As cures for everything from toothaches to acne; aromatherapy and even taken internally for whatever reason is popular that day.. To our own peril, we've discovered much of this information is false. Dr. Turner gains our trust immediately with his treatise: Never ingest these essential oils. And that's the beginning of an author/reader relationship that will stand the test of time…and information, because Dr. Turner tells the truth. And that's the way we like it!

Quit Smoking Naturally

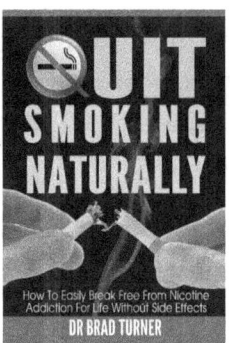

On every literary corner, there's an expert on how to quit smoking. But very few of their theories stick. Every day the weary smoker is inspired to quit, only to have his/her hopes dashed yet again.*Quit Smoking Naturally* is the book that may set everyone free! The genius of this book is the straightforward approach and authentic voice that provides the facts, dispels the fallacies and motivates the smoker to do what they've never done before—succeed at quitting!

The Adrenal Fatigue Cure

The average person knows little about adrenal fatigue let alone where the adrenal glands are located on the body. Situated above the kidneys, these glands, if not working properly, can hinder the function of all the other organs in the body. ADRENAL FATIGUE is an exemplary guide to the adrenal glands—from the symptoms of malfunctioning glands, to adrenal fatigue, even providing an easy to follow diet of delicious foods and beverages that will lead to healthy adrenal glands. ADRENAL FATIGUE should be in every home library. Get your copy today and start the journey to incredible health!

Oil Pulling Therapy The Beginner's Guide

Oil pulling has been around since ancient times but very few people know about this excellent way to oral health and detoxification. This book dispels the myths of oil pulling and gives evidence of its ancient existence and effectiveness. From choosing the oils, to the actual process of pulling, Dr. Brad Turner walks the reader through each step with clarity and simplicity.

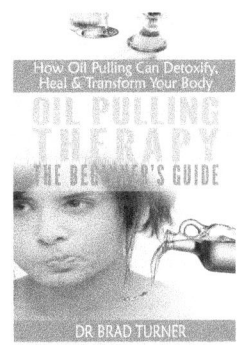

www.ingramcontent.com/pod-product-compliance
Lightning Source LLC
Chambersburg PA
CBHW070235290526
45789CB00004B/1633